Made in the USA
Monee, IL
20 May 2021

69103608R00063